Table of Contents

Adaptive Exercises for Asthma

1. Introduction to Asthma and Exercise

1.1. Understanding Asthma

1.2. Benefits of Exercise for Asthma Management

2. Principles of Adaptive Exercise

2.1. Safety Precautions

2.2. Gradual Progression

3. Types of Adaptive Exercises

3.1. Cardiovascular Exercises

3.2. Strength Training

3.3. Flexibility and Breathing Exercises

4. Adaptive Exercise Programs

4.1. Designing a Personalized Program

4.2. Sample Exercise Routines

5. Monitoring and Adjusting Exercise Intensity

5.1. Using Heart Rate Monitors

5.2. Recognizing Signs of Overexertion

6. Incorporating Adaptive Exercises into Daily Routine

6.1. Home-Based Exercises

6.2. Exercise in Different Environments

7. Psychological Aspects of Exercise for Asthma

7.1. Motivation and Goal Setting

7.2. Coping Strategies for Exercise-Induced Anxiety

8. Nutritional Considerations for Exercise and Asthma

8.1. Balanced Diet for Optimal Performance

8.2. Hydration and Electrolyte Balance

9. Technology and Tools for Monitoring Asthma and Exercise

9.1. Mobile Apps and Wearable Devices

9.2. Peak Flow Meters

10. Research and Evidence-Based Practices in Adaptive Exercise

10.1. Recent Studies and Findings

10.2. Best Practices in Exercise Prescription

Asthma-Friendly Exercises: Strategies and Recommendations

1. Introduction to Asthma and Exercise

2. Understanding Asthma Triggers

3. Benefits of Exercise for Asthma Management

4. Guidelines for Exercising with Asthma

5. Types of Asthma-Friendly Exercises

5.1. 1. Low-Impact Cardiovascular Exercises

5.2. 2. Strength Training

5.3. 3. Flexibility and Breathing Exercises

6. Tips for Exercising Safely with Asthma

6.1. 1. Warm-Up and Cool Down

6.2. 2. Monitoring Your Breathing

6.3. 3. Having a Plan for Emergencies

7. Creating an Asthma-Friendly Exercise Routine

7.1. 1. Setting Realistic Goals

7.2. 2. Tracking Your Progress

8. Conclusion and Final Recommendations

Adaptive Exercises for Asthma

1. Introduction to Asthma and Exercise

Exercise continues to cause a spectrum of symptoms for others because of the narrowing of airways accompanying it. To limit these symptoms, people tend to participate through an adaptive mechanism in the exercises to lower the airway narrowing associated with it. In recent years, because this type of event has developed further, it has led to an increase in evidence criteria to support them and to include the hallmark criteria of either asthma or exercise-induced bronchospasm as a medication on which treatment makers can rely. In some occasions, it sometimes appears inadequate to categorize an individual as an asthmatic or non-asthmatic, but one who has mostly exercise-induced bronchoconstriction, which this article specifically addresses, better corresponds to it.

Introduction: Asthma is a common disease characterized by airway inflammation and large airway hyper-responsiveness. Its common symptoms, occurring in the form of recurrent wheezing, coughing, dyspnea, and chest tightness, take a toll on daily life. The condition also leads to increased airway resistance. Exercise, as a natural stimulator of breathing, can lead to difficult symptoms in most individuals ranging from 40% to 95% and hence, such patients might limit or avoid exercising to avoid these symptoms. Other types of exercise, on the other hand, can improve cardiorespiratory fitness and are associated with a better self-reported quality of life in asthma. As such, people with symptoms of asthma commit themselves to regular physical activity at vigorous intensity.

1.1. Understanding Asthma

It has been reported that the three most common trigger factors of asthma are physical exhaustion, airway cooling, and the inhalation of cold or dry air, including hyperventilation. Doing physical activity with asthma ranges over a wide spectrum from protective to provocative and can result in interruptions of exercise. Despite the high prevalence of asthma, there is currently no cure. Most treatments aim to control the symptoms of the disease by reducing inflammation and relieving bronchial obstruction caused by contractions of smooth muscles in the airways. Nevertheless, studies have repeatedly found that those asthmatics who are inactive or sedentary have a higher risk of having exacerbations than those who are active.

Asthma is a chronic inflammatory disease of the respiratory airways that is characterized by excessive mucus production, bronchospasm, and pulmonary inflammation. This causes repeated episodes of breathlessness, wheeze, sudden cough, and chest tightness. It is estimated that approximately 300 million people are affected by asthma globally, and that the prevalence of asthma is increasing, particularly among children and young adults. Asthma is generally managed through proper treatment, knowing the symptoms and triggers, and visiting a healthcare provider regularly. Education also plays a critical factor in managing asthma. Behavioral strategies include self-management approaches (for example, recognizing and preventing possible triggers, understanding the effects of the medications being taken) and developing peak performance and fitness levels.

1.2. Benefits of Exercise for Asthma Management

Exercise is an important part of managing asthma and maintaining an overall healthy lifestyle. Research shows that in people who follow a daily exercise routine, asthma symptoms are better managed. Although exercise does not appear to improve lung function, it definitely helps to improve other aspects. These might include better quality of life, less psychological distress, improving mood, losing weight, or getting fitter and stronger actually help an individual with asthma to feel better. It can also help decrease the impulse to cough. Overall, research and the opinion of both health professionals and individuals indicate that exercise can be beneficial for those suffering from asthma. Today, most physical therapists working with individuals with asthma would include exercise as part of a treatment program. The nature and amount of exercise would be tailored to individual needs and undertaken on an individual basis.

Exercise combined with other therapies (for example, physiotherapy and medication) can also help with recovery from any flare-ups or asthma attacks.

A well-structured exercise program can be very beneficial for individuals. For asthma management, some of the potential benefits of appropriate regular physical activity include: - more effective breathing pattern - increased fitness - improved mental health - better management of stress, therefore fewer or less severe asthma attacks -

increased energy levels - improved muscle strength and better control of coughing - improved sleep

2. Principles of Adaptive Exercise

Adaptive sessions begin with a general warm-up of the upper body that lasts approximately 15 minutes before specific games or activities chosen by the physiotherapist. Exercises at this level also give the asthmatic time to become familiar with the games. The exercise can be reduced in intensity by, for example, the physiotherapist allowing rest periods. The training program then begins with moderate intensity, and the physiotherapist allocates the training time to the four exercise intensity levels (warm-up, mild intensity, moderate intensity, and vigorous). The exercises at each stage are designed to vary the optimal intensity performed throughout the training time as related to the individual's VT/VEmax.

The quality of life of asthmatic individuals is known to be significantly lower in terms of performing aerobic exercises when compared with healthy individuals of the same age. Therefore, it seems that asthma has negative effects on the cardiovascular system, which can limit physical activity, and decreasing physical activity may increase dyspnea and exacerbation of asthma. Furthermore, in addition to medications, physical therapy and rehabilitation services play a role in the treatment of asthma as non-pharmacological treatments. For this reason, various improvements have been reported in the use of breathing physical therapy or regular and moderate-intensity exercise programs in asthmatic individuals. Therefore, exercise should become a part of the individual's life from the earliest age, and performing personalized exercise will enable more beneficial results to be obtained when compared to pharmacological treatment. For individuals with asthma, adaptive exercises implemented by physiotherapists should be organized with new protocols, but it is not known when to initiate exercises and when to begin exercise with increased intensity.

2.1. Safety Precautions

C. Although compelling data are not available in asthma, joint attention could be paid to primary prevention (preventing the development of the bronchoconstricting response) and secondary prevention (interrupting the chain of events in the asthmatic individual, which lead up to the bronchoconstricting response). At their respective weakest links, interventions may have similar key points: educate about individual risk factors and triggers, optimize the status of co-existing conditions (allergic rhinitis, gastroesophageal reflux, etc.), diminish infectious burden, wear a mask, repair upper airway defects such as septal deviations, silent sinus syndromes, and saddle noses, encourage patients to not talk, sing, or play reeds, have an asthma action plan that tells the patient when and how to take medications, have matching of medication type to individual needs, and maintain rescue therapy. In primary prevention, there may also be a role for consideration of avoidance or diminishment of family members with allergies (but this must be done with extreme caution and may not be ethical in ethics committee settings) absent a long-term double-blinded study showing that watching two cats and three dogs in a house all day every day decreases allergic response, e.g., a direct assessment of causation between pet exposure and allergic sensitization/asthma being low at this time without data for other primary prevention interventions.

B. The acute severity of an attack can be gauged by a pulse rate of > 100 per minute in both children and adults. This condition either requires medical intervention or further reduction of exercise and/or more frequent use of a beta-agonist until recovery occurs.

A. In brief, the young child or older adult with uncontrolled nighttime or early morning attacks may be receiving insufficient long-acting bronchodilator. In this case, a shorter bronchodilator might supplement the control medication at times of greatest need.

2.2. Gradual Progression

In exercise prescription, following the clinical evaluation, the patient's maximal aerobic power (VO2max) may be used as a guide for determining intensity. Assessment of the VO2 max is often difficult for physicians who do not belong to sports medicine or active asthma research. For the need to monitor, consider estimation from the following protocol, which is gradually increased from three periods of physical activity per week. It should be enough to improve the ability to endure the exercise in a safe way. Exercises should be gradual with adequate intervals for rest. We also allow for a cooling period of 15-20 min every time the patient performs exercise, and regular rest during physical activity. If it is the patient's ability, there is no complaint from physical activity up to 30 min. We usually add increments of 5 min per week to 40 min twice. When the patient can last 40 min per period without complaints, we usually increase the intensity according to the Borg score.

Exercise training represents a series of transitions and systematic adaptations made by adopting task-specific physiological demands. This is directly related to increased exercise capacity, so there has to be a gradual increase in either work or intensity. Exercise capacity is determined by ventilatory limitation, diffusion limitation, cardiovascular limitation, and muscular limitation. In asthma, the ventilatory capacity can be affected by bronchospasm which usually manifests as exercise-induced bronchospasm (EIB). As a typical feature in asthma, one common approach to overcoming bronchospasm is preventing bronchoconstriction before exercise.

3. Types of Adaptive Exercises

Breathing exercises: - Belly breathing - Pursed lip breathing - Rib stretches - Deep breathing - Exhaling longer than you inhale

Flexibility (stretching) exercises: - Pulleys, bands and tubing - Yoga - Pilates - Static (or 'traditional') stretches - Stretching using a towel or strap to pull a muscle into stretch

Strength (resistance) training: - Bands and tubes (light) for legs and arms - Light free weights for legs and arms (2 pounds or less) - Machines with weight stack (set between 1 and 3) - Body weight (sit to stand/squats, simple pushups, etc.)

Cardiovascular training (increases the heart rate over a consistent time): - Walking - Biking - Skating or Rollerblading - Aquatic exercises - Rowing - Dancing

Following are a few examples of each type of adaptive exercise that may be suitable for some patients with breathing difficulties.

Individuals who have asthma can enjoy involvement in physical activities just as long as they are attentive and aware of their breathing. There are several different kinds of exercises that can enhance fitness levels, provide enjoyment, and help keep your body functioning well. Professionals agree that incorporating a diversity of exercises into a fitness regimen is the most effective approach. This includes cardiovascular as well as strength and flexibility training. In addition, some people find Pilates beneficial.

3.1. Cardiovascular Exercises

The resistance caused by cardiovascular exercises is based on the nature of various works such as walking, running, and other forms of working. Cardiovascular exercises are a kind of exercise that reduces our body fat and is dissipated in the form of energy. In asthma, individuals generally carry out cardiovascular exercises that require oxygen. Various kinds of exercises are mainly useful in involving cardiovascular training, i.e., walking, jogging, skipping or jumping, and running. By way of normal or deep respiration, cardiovascular exercises increase the strength of the respiratory system or physical inspiration and expiration, helping in the expansion of the lungs and increasing the functional capacity of respiration.

Asthma is actually a condition in which we find difficulty breathing. The word "integrating" in our sentences is due to the situation when our muscles require a constant supply of oxygen regularly for long durations. Oxygen required for our muscles is provided by the air inside us. One study states that unlike healthy individuals, asthma individuals have low endurance capacities to carry out specific work. These asthmatic problems in asthma patients who move from different areas of the house to the bathroom episode are known as cardiovascular exercises in simple elevation. All individuals with asthma must do cardiovascular exercises to improve respiratory functions, even if we have weak resistance, low-endurance capacity, or above-average endurance capacity. It increases the strength of the blood circulatory organs and utilizes oxygen to our maximum capacity.

3.1. Cardiovascular Exercise

3.2. Strength Training

3.2. Strength Training Regular muscle training may help improve the overall fitness of a person with asthma. Strong muscles offer better stability and may help decrease the degree of airway limitations during an asthma exacerbation. Isometric muscle training (e.g., strength and endurance training) for the arms or legs done at the highest intensity that can be tolerated, along with the usual care, can improve strength and endurance in adults with stable moderate to severe asthma. Stronger muscles may help to support breathing in people with asthma. Various types of strength training exercises include free weights, machine weights, bands, balls, and body weight, where all will increase muscle strength to some degree. Borg et al. conducted four weeks of specific inspiratory and expiratory muscle training in adults with severe asthma and found significant increases in inspiratory and expiratory muscle strength compared to the control group, with the greatest difference seen at four weeks. In addition, some emerging research has suggested that the resistance training of lower-limb muscles could reduce symptoms and improve exercise capacity in people with chronic obstructive pulmonary disease. A recent randomized control trial confirmed that specific knee extensor strength training could reduce some asthma symptoms and improve quadriceps endurance.

Respiratory muscle strength is improved by the practice of specific physical exercise, as demonstrated in the details of this guideline. Pre- and post-tests respiratory strength training and other recent publications clearly prove the significance of muscle strength improvement in asthma control.

3.3. Flexibility and Breathing Exercises

One of the problems among patients with persistent asthma is impaired respiratory function, as measured by reduced pulmonary volumes. Decreased pulmonary volume capacity can also have a restrictive impact on physical performance, while flexibility exercises focusing on these pulmonary regularities may help to improve their function as well as the active expiratory muscles. Stretching of muscles, e.g. of the thorax, using flexibility exercises may also prevent dynamic hyperinflation, which otherwise results in increased elastic load and breathing effort. In addition to the positive effects on respiratory function, a reduction in thoracic and bladder stiffness leads to subjective sensations of dyspnea, especially after discontinuation of inspiration. This has been associated with a relaxation effect, as deep breathing helps to calm down. Researchers found vibration and respiratory exercises may be useful as an intervention in the presence of uncontrolled asthma or asthma symptoms. Flexibility exercises seem to provide a useful supplementation in asthma management in both a methodological and practical context.

Current asthma guidelines report evidence of beneficial effects among patients from flexibility as well as breathing exercises. Flexibility exercises, as recommended in many physical activity guidelines, focus on stretching the major muscle groups using slow, gradually increasing movements. Besides the direct effects of improved flexibility, exercises of this type are also recommended for their relaxation effects. Breathing exercises traditionally aim at lowering respiratory frequency or, beneficial specifically for those with EIB, enhance heat and moisture exchange, as discussed in EIB.

4. Adaptive Exercise Programs

We could propose an alternative approach in the design of an adaptive exercise program resulting in a personalized exercise "dosage" directed for reaching the highest FEV1 change without a significant increase in EIB. A feasible personalized asthma adaptive exercise program may be individualized using basic PM diagnosis with an inflammatory kinetics-oriented strategy. An intensity adapted to the individual's energetic demands and driven by the submaximal avoid cold air IETEE tailored in two options (20 or 80 w) is suggested. Such intervention and 6-week home-based rehabilitation program appears to be useful after a period of 1057 3 days of hospital admission to children with intermittent asthma, alleviating bronchial obstructive reversibility by decreasing the EIA positivity rate in week-visit sessions.

A novel approach could be the development of specified indicators for asthma light diagnostically. The asthma kinetics attributes received by monitoring the children over a longer period were used to design an adaptive procedure. A program based on individualized exercise drew on changes in induced sputum cytology during the two initial kinetization flights. The FEV1 reached at the seventh minute of a constant exercise increased to 92% and 85% of initial after intervention and hospital admission, respectively. The stepwise amelioration and possible determination of the beneficial exercise dose based on the individual's inflammatory kinetics and related early functional airway changes could well provide a more effective therapeutic strategy for the children population with asthma. 1-10-1. 10-3-1. 1-10-3. 2-1-2. 2-1-12. 2-1-3.

4.1. Designing a Personalized Program

Adaptive physical activity for asthmatics takes into consideration what the person can or cannot do without affecting the state of his/her asthma management or exacerbations of asthma. The plan may also take into account the season and place of exercise, nature of activity, the need for reliever drugs or lack of it, the site of airway inflammation, or need for symptomatic drugs (if asthma is symptomatic) and exercise-induced bronchoconstriction; developmental stages of the child because currently available drugs can affect the developmental milestones. Young children may feel comfortable playing in water. An adolescent may feel embarrassed if there are too many children around the pool or gym. We have been able to design a special program according to these factors and exercise can be performed in some children. All these activities need relatively moderate intensity exercise. The preventive as well as therapeutic effect are summarized in Table 1. It has been shown by physical therapists over and over that in chronic disease, the single most important factor that consistently predicts long-term success is a regular and appropriate exercise program.

It is considered that some degree of individualization is needed in designing the exercise program. Previous exercise history, fitness level, injuries, available exercise machines, goals of exercise, flexibility to perform exercise in controlled environment, trained personnel to monitor the program and, most importantly, current state of asthma must be evaluated before designing the exercise program for the individual. A twenty year old could run full marathons and then became asthmatic and since then could not run more than 100 metres. Another person could have grade 1 asthma; has never exercised but wants to perform the routine activities without stopping or having symptoms. Another could have no symptoms of asthma but lungs show evidence of it and finds it difficult to exercise unless he/she is with people with a similar problem. These three kinds of exercise activities and need can be met by different exercise programs. Because these people have different symptoms of asthma; the diagnosis, symptoms, quality of life etc., they will also be different. These activities can also be performed in controlled environment.

Friday's Routines A and B Routine B Warm-up: 5-10 minutes Ankle pumps/toe raises: 3 X 20-30 Cool-down: 5-10 minutes

Friday's Routines A and B Routine A Warm-up: 5-10 minutes Ankle pumps/toe raises: 3 X 20-30 Straight leg raises: 3 X 20-30 Cool-down: 5-10 minutes Aerobic

Thursday's Routines A and B Routine B Warm-up: 5-10 minutes Straight leg curls: 2 X 10-15 Ankle pumps: 3 X 20-30 Cool-down: 5-10 minutes Aerobic

Thursday's Routines A and B Routine A Warm-up: 5-10 minutes Straight leg curls: 2 X 10-15 Ankle pumps: 3 X 20-30 Cool-down: 5-10 minutes Aerobic

Tuesday Routine Strength Training Warm-up Aerobic Exercise

Monday's Routines A and B Routine B Warm-up: 5-10 minutes Ankle pumps/toe raises: 3 X 20-30 Cool-down: 5-10 minutes Aerobic

Monday's Routines A and B Routine A Warm-up: 5-10 minutes Ankle pumps/toe raises: 3 X 20-30 Straight leg raises: 3 X 20-30 Cool-down: 5-10 minutes Aerobic Exercise

The following are some example written routines that include a warm-up, 2-3 exercises, and a cool down. The strength training exercise should be performed with little or no resistance at least three times per week. The duration of each routine ranges between 20 – 40 minutes. The aerobic exercise listed should be performed at a moderate to mild intensity for at least 20 minutes or as tolerated. Patients may choose to perform both resistance and aerobic exercises together after the warm up and prior to the cool-down.

5. Monitoring and Adjusting Exercise Intensity

- Ensure the patient isn't overworking with inspiration cycle breathing (dawn of respiration). A significant increase in intensity should cause a noticeable increase in ease of inspiration. - Inspiratory wheel resistance should allow full duration for cycling. - Reducer meter will gradually improve and become closer to expiratory endurance (the patient may show >1/2 expiratory modifier and <1/2 inspiratory modifier). - The majority of the increasing work will relate to inspiratory muscle endurance.

This equation can be the starting point for recommendations about beginning a safe and effective exercise in a child with asthma. Exercise programs for children with exercise-induced asthma that require vigorous (approximating 75% of estimated maximum heart rate) are not likely useful for children with mild EIA. One far easier method for daily control and adjustment is the modified Borg or Children's Exertional Dyspnea Scale. This practical descriptor of perceived symptoms and disability during exercise is illustrated for the reader in Table 6. As the patient's exercise tolerance increases, the exercise intensity should also be increased and vice versa. Adjustment of intensity will depend on the patient's response to exercise testing as well as close observation of training, as increasing training may unmask symptoms that were not present during testing. Following are a few rules of thumb to determine training intensity:

Monitoring and adjusting exercise intensity: Many older protocols for asthma management included the recommendation for using a percentage of predicted maximum heart rate as a gauge for overexerting pediatric patients. Given practical limitations to establishing actual maximal heart rates for pediatric patients, sound clinical guidance has used a workable equation to predict maximum HR in children: estimated maximum HR = 220 - age. All formulae can only be indicative and the response to exercise should be evaluated on an individual basis.

5.1. Using Heart Rate Monitors

Regular aerobic physical exercise can improve exercise capacity by alleviating exercise limitation. The amount of exercise influences physiological improvement. It is important to monitor the exercise intensity of persons with asthma. Heart rate is traditionally used to guide exercise intensity. The heart rate (HR) reflects the response of the cardiovascular system in normal non-asthmatic people as well as the work of breathing in asthmatic adults. Increased ventilation causes elevated oxygen uptake during training with insufficient supplementation of oxygen in patients with fund resistance, thus facilitating higher levels of heart rate. The frequency of heart rate can be a factor in monitoring exercise intensity in individuals with exercise-invoking asthma, and also as a follow-up tool to regulate exercise.

It is useful to monitor the exercise intensity for individuals suffering from asthma. A heart rate (HR) monitor may guide exercise intensity. Heart rate reflects the response of an individual's cardiovascular system to unimproved airflow limitation. Normally, an increase in exercise intensity is followed by a direct increment in exercise heart rate. With a load increase of 1 watt, heart rate may rise 11-14 beats/min. Interval exercises are found to be effective against limited exercise capacity in asthmatic patients. According to the study, the aerobic exercise loads were based on intensities at the anaerobic threshold (AT). To validate such a methodology, we have combined AT loads with heart rate recording to better adjust workloads during "one versus one" interval exercises for men and women with non-steroid-dependent mild-to-moderate asthma. The HR data were analyzed in this paper.

5.2. Recognizing Signs of Overexertion

As with asthma, exercise predisposes individuals with asthma to bronchoconstriction and needed adaptations in breathing to maintain exercise. Classification of asthma severity should include physical wellness and its relationship to mental well-being, the equal part to mental wellness. Severe asthma symptoms might also cause a variety of effects: potentially negatively affecting patient adherence during physical fitness improvement, like regular exercise. Asthma episodes, along with medications or treatments, increase the risk of risk due to severe symptoms of asthma. Passive physical testing protocols would decrease utilization of energy and continual activity during each rest period and produce higher asthma symptoms. If the exercising subject is not allowed extra rest due to overexertion, have increased dosing of rescue beta-agonist medication, and have bronchoconstriction, measure lung function. Adding this measurement should be conducted in conjunction with a health professional. How asthma affects an individual during physical activity for each contribution should be.

Clinical guidance emphasizes recognizing signs of overexertion during activity engagement, including during exercise in asthma. If someone shows visible signs of overexertion – from their face turning red, to their inability to talk, to the pitch of their breathing – they are unable to control their signs of difficulty breathing and they should cease or modify their activity. A guideline for physical activities for people with varying stages and symptoms of asthma has not been developed; however, adaptive physical activity recommendations (e.g., sports, yoga) can be found. Adaptive, patient-led exercises not only reduce the impact of asthma symptoms on physical wellness, but impact the mental wellness as well.

6. Incorporating Adaptive Exercises into Daily Routine

Suggested Adaptive Exercises: 6.1 Exercise due to daily routine: For walking: Taking digital gadgets or putting them in the pockets of your trousers/dress is necessary since walking with empty hands is not realistic for children/teens at present. Taking an essential product like a smartphone gives an equal amount of weight to both sides of the body, which is a low-intensity working two-sided task that assists in balancing both legs, particularly for individuals who fail to balance during static and dynamic activities. This derives two advantages: they get used to waking their wrists to carry something in their hands, such as textbooks, notebooks, stationery, gadgets, and water, without any grip, and the body feels lighter while transferring from two hands to set down because the same weight has been held by both hands.

It's important to discuss how we can instruct individuals who desire to obtain the benefit of adaptation to carry out balance exercises in practical terms. Suggestions for adaptive exercises make more sense when it comes to home-based exercises. There are several activities for adapting to everyday life that need to be conducted under a variety of environmental circumstances, such as exercise while eating, exercising while concentrating on different cognitive activities, or changing indoor and outdoor environments. Adaptive exercises are essential and efficient in all rehabilitation programs, including youth, although particularly in the home, during the COVID-19 pandemic and during periods of adverse weather.

6.1. Home-Based Exercises

Using a few minutes run-up, home-based physical activities can be an efficacious moment of prevention for many patients with asthma that are concentrating mainly on working control. Since even a few minutes of "do what you can" can check exercise capacity and correct the subjects if this is impaired, there is the need for simple and standardized few minutes indoor tests in asthma management. Therefore, exercise and health professionals should promote the practice of unplanned but regularly repeated and regular "do what you can" physical activities in patients with asthma. Historically, exercise was considered a contraindication for children with asthma. Regular physical activity is associated with improved exercise-induced asthma, increased airway caliber, greater antioxidant defenses, and reduced perception of dyspnea during exercise.

For an improvement in asthma control, adults are now being advised to participate regularly in at least 150 minutes (2½ hours) of moderate-intensity or at least 75 minutes (1¼ hours) of vigorous-intensity aerobic and muscle-strengthening activities on 2 or more days a week. However, most individuals with asthma do not meet these exercise recommendations and have a sedentary way of life. Although benefits have been described from systematic physical activity on health and regulation of the immune system, each season many data show that the descent of degree asthma control could be related to reduced physical activity, even in people with intermittent and mild asthma. It is also impossible for the majority of patients to train in the gym because of distance, difficulty parking, not enough time, and inconvenience.

There are many public areas that are used for exercise, such as tracks, gymnasiums, swimming pools, and other areas where there is space. Individuals with asthma exercise in all of these environments. Many people participate in groups to exercise, or they may have individual programs to follow. This provides the ability to tailor an individual patient's exercise to the environment that may be safer for them. This assists in the prescription of exercise and individual exercises for patients with asthma. There are new types of exercise classes that are being run in the community and are designed for groups of patients with asthma. They include tai chi, yoga, and some cardiovascular training classes where patients can use a spinning bike and portable inspiration devices (pMDIs packaged inside vacuum-shimmed spacers).

When we talk about exercise in the environment, it usually means exercising outside of the normal environment. The normal environment in a community is usually a family house where asthma patients do the majority of their exercise. If the patient can exercise more without asthma symptoms in another environment, we can possibly adjust an exercise program to their activity level based on it. For example, during pollen season, going to a shopping mall or laser play can reduce the amount of pollen exposure. In these cases, we should suggest that the patient try exercising in these environments. On the other hand, for an asthmatic patient, going to a night club can be an area of exposure to irritants such as passive smoking and perfumes. Therefore, it may not be appropriate to exercise in this environment.

7. Psychological Aspects of Exercise for Asthma

It is crucial that physiotherapists possess specific strategies for promoting participation in home exercise during asthma, many of which have application across chronic conditions in general. Aspects which are relevant to the promotion of exercise during asthma are likely to include a degree of physical discomfort when exercising, embarrassment at having heart and breathing rates exceeded by others, and simple physical adaptations to exercise. Ultimately, in order that exercise may be carried out safely and effectively at home, those with asthma need to have a repertoire of skills, knowledge, and resources which enable them to balance their enjoyment of exercise with an ability to recognize symptoms of overexertion.

An extensive body of opinion supports the view that appropriate participation in physical activity is relevant to the psychological well-being of the individual. Lifestyle-related activities are an important source of sociality and affiliated person satisfaction and fulfillment; a circumstance which is particularly relevant in the context of exercise in asthma. Exercise in asthma is central to the adoption of a curriculum aimed at improving the quality of life through the enhancement of and the maintenance of a degree of physical fitness acceptable to the asthmatic person. Psychological problems must be addressed and support must be provided in the form of coping strategies. The problem of exercise-induced anxiety must be addressed specifically while emphasis should be placed on enhancement of psychosocial factors. Above all, each person's individual needs and desires should be taken into account and addressed. In the production of an exercise prescription, this aspect will be covered when speaking about goal setting and motivation.

7.1. Motivation and Goal Setting

Exercise can be very daunting, at the best of times, and goals and motivation can be a hindering factor. In someone with asthma or COPD, effective goal-setting and motivation will be key for adopting and maintaining an adaptive exercise plan. As an example, someone with asthma may avoid exercise if they are constantly focused on their personal best, join a gym, do HIIT and run 5K's. It is well documented that greater symptoms are experienced at higher intensities of exercise via an increased minute ventilation, resulting in cooler and drier air being brought into the airways. However, parents and patients in my clinics more often than not want their treatment plan in an A4 piece of paper with bullets. Base-level information does not cover why exercising in certain ways is detrimental to one's health. For example, a patient should learn about not doing excessive exercise when they have had a cold because the load on the cardio-respiratory system when exercising at a high intensity could promote bronchoconstriction as the warm humidified breathing volume increases.

Research has shown that asthma can be exacerbated by exercise. However, there is an extensive body of work that has shown that exercise can be highly beneficial to individuals with asthma. In view of this, psychologists are increasingly being included in interdisciplinary teams to help people who are sedentary adopt a more healthy lifestyle. This requires their physical health to be at a level that it currently is not and overcoming a psychopathology, e.g. overcoming a fear of movement or fear of asthma exacerbation.

7.2. Coping Strategies for Exercise-Induced Anxiety

Compiled from Rabe, K.F. and Knotter, J., Exercise-Induced Airway Obstruction: A Disabling Disease, and Whodunit? Asthma. Schattauer, New York, pp. 154-160, 1994, Rec: 4.

Giving the new patient a "No choice"/Just do it attitude may reflexly counter physical conditioning. In fact, patients may correct you by saying, "Doctor, I still can't do it." This type of dialogue perpetuates psychological holding-on. Psychologically, a patient feels powerful when he/she has others hold him/her back from doing something. Keep in mind; sticking with exercise "aggravates" the muscle tissue at the same time (early on) the asthmatic airways, thus sending inaccurate messages to the "fight-or-flight mechanism" - you either reduce the amount of exercise or wait, if you are wrong, you lose.

7.2.1 Helping with Exercise Strategy: Just do it ("No Choice...")

Each program has group sessions lasting 30 minutes with the remaining 30 minutes of scheduled exercise to practice planned coping strategies. The psychologist is assigned the responsibility to ensure exercise is conducted with the assigned coping strategy. Subsequent to participation in the program, the subjects were questioning fund of knowledge for lifestyle exercise activities and reported time being more relaxed in approach to activity.

Coping with exercise-induced asthma through lifestyle changes can be stressful to the individual with asthma. In part, exercise is inferred to be good physically and psychologically. Tradition and current literature imply that exercise is fun and if it were not, no one would do it except for the very few fierce competitors. The assumption is made that once the fun, enjoyment, and quality of life derived from exercise is known, the individuals will get outside and play without ever mentioning it. This is a valid assumption since the vast majority of information and discussion at large focuses on opportunities or the positives of exercise.

The personal strategies for coping with challenges associated with physical activities are varied: clear communication of physical limitations to others involved in an exercise program; belief that their need for fast relief medications outweighs the good they might experience with exercise - intimidated by the duration of action with long-term use of medications; enjoyed the life of ease and did not wish to add further chores to the day; were influenced by their health professionals' attitude that exercise may cause harm; became too out of shape to exercise without experiencing great difficulty; the severity of their asthma precluded them from attempting to workout - fearing that they would become panic-stricken and/or need immediate medical attention which would be difficult to obtain.

Individuals who struggle with an activity often walk away physically, but the psychological effects of not being able to cope with whole body exercise linger longer than the discomfort of asthma associated with exercise. The one question every patient with asthma asks is, "Why me?" When facing exercise-induced asthma, the question probably becomes "Why exercise?" The fears and doubts associated with asthma symptoms induced by exercise could be enough to limit the person to a sedentary lifestyle.

Abstract Subsection 7.2: Coping Strategies for Exercise-Induced Anxiety

8. Nutritional Considerations for Exercise and Asthma

Adaptive exercise incorporating components of inspiration and expiration could conceivably change the mechanics and neural coordination of the airways and reduce EIA. While evidence of this effect from studies of various airway field sports such as swimming, rowing, and running are equivocal, the asthmatic performing an adaptive exercise in excess of the MAV has the potential to improve endurance performance provided they consume enough oxygen. Nutritional considerations in HNDE are therefore twofold: a well-balanced diet should be consumed to meet the energy needs of exercise with the potential to improve ventilatory function and prevent EIB while maintaining hydration and electrolyte balance.

Good nutrition with a balanced diet provides fuel and nutrients necessary for optimal exercise performance and training adaptation. An additional nutritional issue relevant to individuals with asthma is ensuring adequate fluid intake and maintenance of a balanced hydration state. A diet that supports good general health, which includes a high consumption of fruit and vegetables, whole grains, and sufficient dairy produce, while maintaining a low consumption of saturated and trans fats, has been shown in some studies to reduce the risk of asthma. While this benefit has been linked to the anti-inflammatory effects of consuming omega-3 fatty acids and vitamin D, fatty fish and sun exposure to meet adequate intake may be relatively unpalatable for many people who have asthma. In the authors' opinion, the greater nutritional concern for people with asthma is hydration and ensuring electrolyte balance becomes an exercise adaptation.

8.1. Balanced Diet for Optimal Performance

There is no such class of food that can cure or control asthma, but an asthma patient can have a meal as per the requirement of everyday need. The dietary factors include antioxidants, lipid peroxidation, omega-3, beta-carotene, vitamin C, magnesium, low salt diet, natural salicylates, histamine, and food sensitivities. Physical activity is the behavior of the metabolic machinery and the major user of energy, and it also assures one's health. The nutritional requirement reflects in a person with physical activity and at rest. The metabolism of food should supply energy for muscle action, sustain appetite when coming from practice/training or competition. In sufficient calorie intake stages, low carbohydrate diets are rehearsed in an exercise routine, and that need significantly of stored metabolic fuel. Consequently, good fuel replenishment can affect the athlete's performance and has an impact on day-to-day activity and health. A varied and balanced diet is essential and a nonzero sum game that supports health, energy, and optimal weight, and helps prevent illness and aids recovery in the body. In adjusted equilibrium, certain vitamins and minerals and antioxidants are needed for general health, exercise, and sport. Carbohydrate, protein, fat, and hydration are the most important dietary fuel substances.

Exercising with asthma is a common anxiety feeling. The consequences are various, including wheezing, coughing, chest discomfort, increased mucus production, asthma attack, and exercise-induced bronchoconstriction. In the climax of exercise, a respiratory heat loss appears because of the extraversion from the bronchial capillary bed to the cooling of the inspired air. On inhalation, the intrapulmonary and tracheal airway gets vasoconstricted, and when physical exertion is pushed, intrapulmonary shunt is reflected on nutritionally supported sportsmen. Nutrition and asthma, a link has to be maintained for optimal performance of an asthmatic individual. Asthma is classified as an inflammatory airway disease characterized by bronchial hyper-responsiveness.

8.2. Hydration and Electrolyte Balance

There's conflicting evidence about whether electrolyte repletion might help to damp down EIB in some people. However, maintaining adequate hydration and electrolyte balance in general is crucial for the functioning of basic bodily functions, many of which are critical in helping to manage asthma. Generally, it is thought that individuals who are completing intense exercise sessions in a cool environment, or for more than 4 hours in warmer environments may benefit from adding in sodium to their hydration with fluids or food to help replace sodium losses. At a basic level, the simplest method to monitor this is to aim to consume enough fluid to limit weight loss due to dehydration to less than 2% of body weight in total or serious adverse effects.

Electrolyte balance is a crucial part of exercise performance. Nerves and muscles - including those that expand and contract the lung - depend on the movement of charged ions to transmit information and generate movement. Sodium, potassium, and chloride are particularly important in driving these functions, although other ions also play a supportive role. Dehydration can exacerbate pre-existing exercise-induced bronchoconstriction (EIB). It's thought this happens because of an increased osmotic load in the airway lining fluid: this - in conjunction with an increased airway surface fluid concentration of pro-inflammatory molecules - is thought to encourage movement of water out of the cell and into the airway lumen where it will react with the high salt concentration in the sweat. This can trigger osmotic stress, leading to increased nerve firing and reflex narrowing of the airway. Although this isn't asthma, it could contribute to the severity of asthma.

As a person with exercise-induced asthma, it is often recommended to ensure you are staying well-hydrated during exercise. This is good advice, but the reason behind this isn't usually given. In this short section, we briefly delve into the biology of hydration and electrolyte balance, and give some practical advice on how to maintain this balance.

9. Technology and Tools for Monitoring Asthma and Exercise

Peak flow meters provide a numerical measurement of lung function and an objective way to determine a patient's best lung function. A peak flow zone is based on your best value. The red zone is 60-39% of your best value, the yellow zone is 80-61% of your best value, and green is 100-81% of your best value. If your peak flow value is in the red zone, this may be an indication of an asthma episode, and you may need to change your action plan or take your bronchodilator according to the asthma action plan. However, peak flow values are generally not accurate values during exercise, as the values can change for a variety of reasons and may be a low or high peak flow. It is important to use symptoms and/or pulse to pair with peak flow values. When combined with exercise, you should monitor your symptoms and/or pulse in addition to your peak flow.

Mobile apps and wearable devices are very popular tools for monitoring and measuring specific exercise intensity while exercising. They are also good tools for tracking step count and calorie expenditure. However, it is important for individuals with asthma to be able to pair or integrate the tracked exercise intensity from mobile apps and wearable devices with their asthma control and symptoms. There are some mobile apps and wearable devices that have been designed specifically for PEF and FEV1 monitoring using a smartphone or digital peak flow meter. You can visit the mobile apps and tools in the coaching course under the exercise and symptom monitoring sections.

9.1. Mobile Apps and Wearable Devices

Many researchers are working on digital relief tools that could improve the health status of adults with asthma, such as mobile apps to monitor air quality and daily physical activity in the neighborhood, built-in smartphone exercise video apps with cost-effective programs, easy-to-follow, and motivational videos, and digital interventions for increasing physical activity using personalized SMS texts and tailored email information. Built-in smartphone tools are easy to integrate, accessible to everyone, and can help in monitoring and managing physical activity. Accessories include smartphone-based mobile sensors and devices and sports cameras. Some of the known smartphone-based popular free apps, like Google Fit or Samsung Health, can track physical activity in real-time, such as walking, running, cycling, and calories burned.

Mobile apps and wearable devices, such as smartphones, smartwatches, and mobile sensors, have been extensively used in various fields and are digital platforms that integrate various solutions. For asthmatics who are engaged in exercise, previous studies have shown an increase in the number of tools to manage physical activity, as well as a need to monitor daily activity. The following subsections review the technological solutions available for persons with asthma to monitor their physical activity level and manage their physical activity. In addition, technological innovation has the potential to help people with asthma adhere to regular exercise and manage their asthma symptoms. By implementing a deep-learning model to evaluate respiratory rate (RR) (a symptom noticed during high-intensity exercise for asthmatics) and classifying different physical activities, the study presented a new concept for developing a single In-house Sensor (IoT sensor) to monitor activity in individuals with asthma.

9.2. Peak Flow Meters

Before Exercise: Peak expiratory flow measurements taken at rest, no earlier than 20 minutes following taking a breathing medication, provide beneficial information. Your peak flow meter will monitor the maximum amount of air you can expel from your lungs (in liters per second) and may be used to record daily peak flow readings during rest or pre/post-exercise therapy. Many physicians help patients to handle their asthma based on their peak flow readings. When exercise occurs, it is reasonable to expect peak flow predictions of 20 to 30 liters per minute.

A peak flow meter is a device used to measure how much air a person can expel from their lungs. Asthma, chronic obstructive pulmonary disease (COPD), or other lung diseases may be detected using this procedure. By comparing how much air the lungs can expel during a slow exhalation, peak flow measurements can also assess airway resistance. For some people with asthma and exercise-induced bronchospasm, keeping an eye on lung function is critical.

Monitoring peak expiratory flow is one of the easiest ways to know if your breathing is on track. You may not be using your peak flow meter correctly. If your doctor has prescribed a peak flow monitor, it's important to understand how to use the device. Watching for results that fall below your personal best (as well as using preventive measures) is critical for managing asthma and exercise-induced bronchospasm. Not only do low readings provide information on how well your medications are working and whether adjustments need to be made, but they also alert you to potential danger.

10. Research and Evidence-Based Practices in Adaptive Exercise

Additional research is needed to examine the mechanisms why different protocols of interval training (both moderate continuous and high-intensity) and comprehensive exercise can have a positive effect both on decreasing the level of eosinophils/neutrophils in peripheral blood and sputum and an increase in response to the use of adenosine diphosphate-induced platelet aggregation; neurotransmitter levels (serotonin, histamine) and transforming growth factor b1 exhaled breath condensate in patients with BA. Practices for prescribing physical training are presented in both international and national practice-oriented documents—medical and athletic. Therefore, the use of these protocols can be recommended to improve the quality of life for all patients with BA and, accordingly, reduce public spending, as passive behavior leads to a decrease in exercise capacity and, therefore, to secondary somatic dysfunctions caused by hypokinesia and not an increase in pulmonary ventilatory dysfunction.

Synopsis: Physical activities can contribute to the overall maintenance of one's well-being and positively affect their physical, mental, and social status. Here, we provide only the most recent scientific data regarding adaptive exercises, adapted gymnastics, adapted swimming, adapted gymnastics for children, adapted sports, and adapted physical education in terms of people with asthma or COPD. Adaptive exercises are part of non-pharmacological treatments in all severity grades of bronchial asthma (BA) and can be carried out both by medical prescription under the supervision of physiotherapists, health professionals, and coaches, as well as independently, under the supervision of a physical education teacher. The latest high-quality systematic reviews prove that practicing exercises has a positive effect on improving the exercise capacity and the health quality of patients with bronchial asthma. Currently, seven national and international guidelines contain the recognized practices for prescribing the adaptive exercises in people with BA, as well as evidence from scientific research.

10.1. Recent Studies and Findings

The question is, how much do we need to do adaptive exercises to improve lung function, immune inflammatory responses, and lung health for asthmatics? Or compare focus time, quantity and optimal sample model to recommend adequate adaptive exercise therapy. Many questions arise as to what kind of adaptive physical activity is recommended in the meanwhile. Therefore, this article was prepared to be able to summarize the findings of recent studies regarding the effects of adaptive exercise therapy programs in improving lung function, the regulation of immune inflammation and the regulation of airway smooth muscle function in patients with asthma. Hopefully therapists therapy can devise advanced asthma on the basis of scientific evidence these papers.

The evidence for exercise-induced bronchoconstriction (EIB) is extensive, but research is still emerging as to the benefit of adaptive exercises for asthmatics. Currently, exercise training with a specific physiological improvement focuses on aerobic capacity, V_E and V_T, oxidative function and the endocrine side of the agreement. However, there are relatively recent, but still very few papers that have proven the benefit of adaptive exercise activities with biological, psychological and anti-inflammatory values for people with asthma, especially the controversial process of the genetic aspects of 'training response'.

10.2. Best Practices in Exercise Prescription

More importantly, there is still a trend in the design of adaptive exercise regimens, citing that the benefits of exercise for people with asthma and exercise-induced bronchoconstriction can be achieved through training regimens of only 8 to 12 weeks in length, with minimal to no attention paid to long-term (1 year or more) programs in the literature. As a result, effective adaptations are minimal, once you consider that some of the longest single-focused free-living environmental studies researching exercise on people with asthma have gone out in trial for a period of 6, 9, and 12 months in length! Researchers have called out, in at least one prior study, for the development of an "exercise prescription model capable of sustained protection through a regular program of physical activity." To date, an evidence-based, long-term, adaptive exercise training tier consisting of flexibility, cardio-resistance, and endurance has yet to be really appreciated in the scientific community.

In order to optimally prescribe exercise for individuals with asthma, it is necessary to know and apply best practices based on the most current and evidence-supported literature. Researchers throughout the world have for decades studied such factors as exercise-induced bronchoconstriction symptoms, reduction in exercise capacity and mortality, inflammation, medications, and many other central points pertaining to the relationships between asthma and exercise. It is essential for professionals around the world to familiarize themselves with this research as best they can and integrate these data into the practice of best practice-based, adaptive exercise session construction. Knowing how to apply such information can translate into initial adaptations and the consistent changes in the exercise prescription, which are major elements of an effective plan in incremental adaptations. The substance of these incremental program adaptations, as well as logging when they were initiated and, to the best of our knowledge, the response to the changes in the exercise prescription, challenge the athlete and support the ACSM AAP as the template for asthma-conditioning program growth.

Asthma-Friendly Exercises: Strategies and Recommendations

1. Introduction to Asthma and Exercise

The following strategies have been helpful to many asthma patients - use them as a part of your asthma active routine if they work for you. It is important to stress, however, that not all of these exercises are safe for every person with asthma. A few recommended starting points may be suggested here, but the best course is for this person to consult with a pulmonary specialist or other physician who is familiar with or has experience with asthma and exercise. Consulting with a professional who knows about both asthma and the best exercises to lose fat (caloric expenditure) will decrease the chances of having your asthma triggered. This way, you'll be able to get a personalized exercise program that accomplishes your weight loss goals, lose the highest body fat percentage, and avoid losing weight in muscle, and also fits your schedule. A careful asthma-friendly exercise plan can also reduce the mucus that's constantly being over-secreted in the lungs of a person with asthma.

While many people may have this lung condition in which the bronchial tubes constrict on a regular basis, not all of these people should have difficulty exercising. Although some might use their asthma as an excuse not to venture out into physical activity, the fact is that carefully designed exercise can benefit both the body and the symptoms of asthma. But because some patterns of physical activity can lead to asthma symptoms, and because having asthma may have other considerations even when exercising does not stimulate these symptoms, it is worthwhile to consider what exercise is safe for the average patient with asthma to engage in. This will give you an idea of what types of activities to choose for a fitness program for the asthma patient. If the person has already chosen activities, you can use this list to help guide the person in how to make these activities less likely to bring on asthma symptoms with helpful techniques for people with asthma.

2. Understanding Asthma Triggers

Always check the air quality report and the weather report before exercising outdoors. Humidity may trigger asthma in some people. Outside activity might best be done when the humidity is low. Air pollution can irritate the lungs and trigger asthma, especially for people who observe their asthma flaring when the air quality index is high. Low pollution areas to jog or walk are wooded trails and parks. Opt for a gym instead of a running path if the oxygen concentration of the air outside is bad.

For some people with asthma, physical activity can be a trigger. Other common asthma triggers include allergens (like pet dander, dust mites, and pollen), respiratory infections, irritants (like smoke, mold, strong odors, and fumes), certain medications, and changes in the weather. Perform different exercises indoors instead of outdoors on high pollen count days. During the winter, the indoor environment is often warm and dry, which can aggravate asthma symptoms. That's why it's extra important to take precautions to avoid an asthma flare-up if you exercise indoors during the winter. For example, cold weather and snow can trigger asthma symptoms in some people. It's always a good idea to layer up, covering your nose and mouth with a scarf and reducing outdoor exercise in the winter to lessen exposure to cold air.

Many people experience asthma symptoms when they exercise. But this doesn't have to stop you from playing sports or doing other activities. By recognizing what triggers your asthma, you can work with your healthcare providers to create an asthma action plan that helps you exercise safely.

3. Benefits of Exercise for Asthma Management

Moreover, regular exercise enhances the strength of the inspiratory muscles and diaphragm. As such, the act of breathing becomes more efficient overall. People with asthma may also use breathlessness during exercise to desensitize their bodies to this feeling. Exercise-induced bronchoconstriction (EIB) might actually be induced by breathing in air that is drier and colder than 37° and its stimulating effect on the nervous system, which cannot be replicated any other way. Aerobic exercise, of the kind steady-state cardio, is the most recommended exercise for people with asthma. Forty minutes of aerobic exercise a day three to five days a week is recommended by the American College of Sports Medicine. However, plenty of home-based approaches exist. To get airborne allergens out of your airways, for example, you can practice blowing up a balloon a few times in a row when you know you are going to exercise the next day. Breath-focused yoga is also very good at boosting voluntary control of the respiratory system and causing bronchodilation. In order to exercise safely, people with asthma should always seek advice from their healthcare provider.

Regular physical activity is good for everyone, whether or not they have asthma. This statement is true for several reasons. First, exercise offers several mental health benefits. In addition, studies have revealed that people with asthma who engage in regular exercise tend to have enhanced lung function compared to those with asthma who lead a sedentary lifestyle. In a 2017 study featuring two hundred and seventy confirmed asthma patients, it was discovered that greater physical activity levels were linked to lower respiratory inflammation biomarkers, such as nitric oxide and IgE antibodies—these levels were even lower in asthma patients who met international physical activity requirements.

4. Guidelines for Exercising with Asthma

The process of writing and implementing an asthma management plan unique to each individual is called collaborative self-management. This method takes a person's unique signs and symptoms, requirements, abilities, and skills into account. Collaboration with a professional healthcare provider can verify the client's beliefs and goals, as well as appraise their lifestyle and the resources available. The main goal of all asthma medications is to control asthmatic symptoms and maintain normal lung function. The main components of an exercise plan include the therapeutic relationship, exploring the client's asthma medication use, assessing client barriers to medication use, partnerships for inhaler skills and technique training, inhaler choice, and a written asthma management action plan. Types of medicines (e.g., reliever as needed for wheeze, preventer medicines for regular exercise induced symptoms, and premedication before exercise) can be explored with clients.

- Determining medical emergency knowledge and management.

- Assessing individual physical activity history assists the instructor in establishing an individualized exercise plan that might include a combination of alternative activities (e.g., walking or swimming) that are less likely to produce EIB.

- Assessing barriers, limitations, and concerns before designing and implementing an individualized exercise program is essential. This should include bronchoconstriction and beta-agonist use related to physical activity, exercise intensity, high-intensity activities, comorbid conditions, and asthma medications used. Also, recommendations will be provided regarding medications in case of severe symptoms.

- Individuals have to obtain medical clearance from a healthcare practitioner prior to beginning an exercise program.

Prior to starting an exercise program, some general guidelines must be carefully considered:

5. Types of Asthma-Friendly Exercises

Many individuals with asthma and those without asthma may engage in strength training. It can be done with hand weights, dumbbells, kettlebells, ankle and wrist weights, resistance bands, bodyweight exercises, or weight machines. Additionally, when an individual is not acutely symptomatic or experiencing a lung infection, they may even increase the intensity to include plyometric exercises. The most benefit is found when completing 2–4 sets of 8–10 different exercises 2–3 days per week.

Asthma and fitness: Although this type of workout will not build strength, endurance, and heart health, it can improve mental health. Whether to exercise indoors or out will depend on each individual's asthma triggers. Keep in mind that environmental conditions vary greatly among different parts of the world. It's important to pace yourself when you do a cardiovascular workout. Don't push yourself to become "out-of-breath," though. This could trigger asthma symptoms and could be dangerous. Use your short-acting inhaler 20 minutes before you start to exercise to prevent symptoms. Wait at least 10 minutes after you're done before you take your breathing treatment, whether you used it before exercise or not. If you don't have an exercise-induced asthma treatment plan, talk to your healthcare provider.

Examples: - Walking - Cycling (preferably in dry air) - Dance - Water aerobics (pool exercise) - Rowing - Cross-country ski machine - Step machines

Low-impact cardiovascular (aerobic) exercises:

There are many types of exercises that are suitable if you have asthma, and participation in regular physical activity may improve fitness in individuals with asthma, in addition to being beneficial for other health conditions. Here's an example of one of the categories of suitable exercises for people with asthma. For more options, see the full article "Physical Activity and Asthma."

5.1. 1. Low-Impact Cardiovascular Exercises

Walking should be introduced to a person who is new to exercise as 5-10 minutes of walking a day warrants a few days of adjustment. Walking programs can then be implemented by increasing time spent exercising by 5-10 minutes after every 7-10-day period, with benefits being realized after a period of 30 minutes exercised a day at least five days per week. Guidelines recommend that a cycle speed of ≥60 revolutions per minute (rpm) be maintained when cycling for 30 minutes, five days a week, to see benefit. Swimming will likely require a progressively slower incremental increase in laps, due to the fact that the movement of swimming may seem easier but the steady contact and resistance the water provide may take a greater initial toll on the body.

Regardless of an individual's level of asthma control, optimal care should be exercised to select exercises and intensities that do not aggravate pre-existing asthma symptoms. As such, low-impact cardiovascular exercises that are easy on the joints and improve cardiovascular fitness without challenging the respiratory system should be introduced for a person who has both asthma and joint pain. Walking, swimming, and cycling are generally good places to begin. These exercises can help to build muscle endurance while sparing the joints due to their low-impact nature. People with asthma who experience decreased ventilatory efficiency and tidal volume with moderate and high-intensity activities may benefit from moderate-intensity activities. While all activities present the same intensity, one 2019 study found that swimming was but one of three activities that afforded subjects the opportunity to achieve the lowest required amount of energy expenditure for the greatest improvement in exercise capacity.

Low-impact cardiovascular exercises

5.2. 2. Strength Training

An alternative to equipment for resistance training is utilizing the body. Another option would be to use the body as resistance. Push-ups, sit-ups, and chin-ups are included in this form of exercise. This does not imply, however, that individuals find it tough to breathe and, because of their asthma, they feel they can handle these kinds of exercises and avoid them. This type of resistance training is not included in respiratory muscular training. It includes lifting weights – no heavy weights. In order to accumulate resistance, the muscles get tired by repeating the action. Strength training should always start with 1-2 sets for each of the exercises and at least 5-10 minutes of warm-ups.

Strength training Individuals restricted by their asthma-associated symptoms, as well as children and adolescents, can benefit from strength training workouts. Enhancing overall strength does not necessarily influence direct training of the breathing muscles, but it can indirectly support excellent performance in endurance activities, particularly in cases of improvement of overall muscle strength in weak muscles. In terms of performing strength training exercises, the following advice should be considered: The movements should be smooth and slow, and only one set of 8-12 repetitions should be performed. In order to get results, the workouts should be conducted as often as possible, with two to three workouts per week. Some routines can often be carried out for those who are relatively fit with serious asthma as long as the medication is properly used. They should never, however, exercise without consulting their doctor and/or respiratory therapist. Options include free weights, such as dumbbells, or weight machines. To limit the weight, resistant bands or tubing bands can be used. Instruction from a professional instructor is recommended.

5.3. 3. Flexibility and Breathing Exercises

Breathing control means that the air will flow to the desired alveolus within the range. Breathing control activities include breathing exercises or retraining of certain diaphragmatic breaths. Specific breathing techniques help people with asthma reduce hyperventilation. We must regulate and slow down the entire breathing process. This technique helps reduce airway resistance due to cooling. available information shows that the combination of yoga and meditation stabilizes asthma. For those who do not have allergies, diaphragmatic smooth yoga breathing can also relax the smooth muscles in the bronchioles.

However, the importance of focusing on this review is that a few people, both in the gold and silver groups, mentioned that breathing exercises were recommended to learn and practice before increasing physical activity, such as power walking. Flexibility is important for any joints and muscles, including the bronchus, diaphragm, intercostals, serratus anterior, and abdominal muscles. One of the key pointers for flexibility is good posture. We can maintain the posture of an individual with asthma through nerve motor system control, stretching, strengthening the diaphragm muscle, and increasing the muscle of the pectoralis sympathetic with respiratory exercises.

During asthma, the respiratory muscles can get tight due to reversible airway obstruction caused by inflammation and hyperresponsiveness, as well as stressful breathing habits.

We can improve flexibility in respiratory muscles in different ways. Yoga and pilates improve the flexibility of respiratory muscles mainly through stretching, relaxation, meditation, mood improvement, and self-care for people with asthma. A focus group interview with people with asthma revealed that not everyone had positive experiences regarding increased quality of life after participating in yoga.

6. Tips for Exercising Safely with Asthma

Remember, communicating with your doctor is very important. He or she can help provide information on recommended routines and avoid potential problems, suggest strategies for safe and beneficial exercise, provide appropriate asthma medications and guidance on the use of asthma medications, and develop an asthma action plan that helps control your asthma. Thirteen percent of athletes diagnosed with exercise-induced asthma are black; therefore, it is also important to consult with your doctor as well. Proper names spaces here are: asthma, black, names, white, windows, Drupal, medical site.

- Begin and end your activity with a warm-up and cool down. - Monitor your breathing pattern as a guide to the intensity of a workout. - Studies show that people who had recently had a severe attack are more likely to suffer an attack during or just after exercising. - If you need a quick-acting inhaled bronchodilator, take it prior to exercising to maintain normal airway function. - If you are subject to exercise-induced asthma, a bronchodilator taken before exercise can decrease the symptoms. - Always have your asthma rescue medication available. - Athletes are encouraged to have their medication nearby during play and make sure the coach or supervisor is familiar with their asthma action plan in case of an emergency. - It's always a good idea to cool down and talk to your doctor when an unexpected or emergency bout of exercise-induced asthma occurs.

Physical activities do a body good; the benefits to our health are numerous. Though individuals with asthma often forgo the practice for fear of an attack or a struggle to breathe once they begin, it is important to note that people living with asthma can and do compete in long distance running, ballet, basketball, and soccer. By following some simple precautions, exercise can be your friend. Here are some tips for practicing safe exercise with asthma:

6.1. 1. Warm-Up and Cool Down

Experts now emphasize the importance of regular physical activity for both health and disease diagnosis. However, for the purpose of exercise with shortness of breath, special attention should be paid to warm-up and cool-down. Some relaxation combined with endurance activity programs does not increase asthma risk. Studies have shown that warming and stretching exercises can have a positive effect on ventilatory function. It can ensure a gradual heart rate per minute and decrease both extra metabolism and the risk of hyperventilation. It also allows muscles to work effectively and in dense weight cases. Because of these benefits, cool-down should not be neglected. A significant factor to take care of during exercise is that, in any case, it must be effective and safe. When exercising with asthma, do not forget this process, which is also important. The need to apply a cool-down period after exercise also shows that the benefits need to be mentioned in terms of the topic even more. With this article, the effects of exercise on asthma will be evaluated and the validity of cooling techniques will be reviewed. In many cases, the relation between exercise-induced asthma and optional add-on drugs will be discussed. Itineraries for rules and regulations where offseason cannot be armed will also be included campaign.

Cooling down exercises are very important. If you are an asthma sufferer, it is also one effective way to monitor how well your asthma is healing, and it can also help you significantly reduce premature asthma symptoms. Loss of flexibility has caused many asthma attacks during exercise. Therefore, you need to supplement some stretching exercises before and after exercising. In many diseases, there is no cure for asthma but instead focuses on the prevention and relief of the severity of asthma symptoms.

6.2. 2. Monitoring Your Breathing

For example, if you start wheezing or coughing while outside running, it is important to slow down and walk for a quick moment to get your breathing back on track. If you are not sure, then try pursed lip breathing for a couple of minutes to see if things improve. In summary, it is well worth the effort to learn how your breathing pattern feels and how it responds to changes in your body. By practicing this asthma-friendly exercise strategy, you are better equipped to tailor your workouts to match your body's needs. One improved aspect of your asthma management is that you reduce or eliminate those out-of-control situations.

Another aspect of self-monitoring involves developing an awareness of your breathing as you exercise. With time, you can learn what your normal breathing pattern looks and feels like while you work out. If you notice that your breathing pattern changes or the effort of your breath becomes more difficult or uncomfortable, you can choose to reduce your exercise intensity to prevent further difficulty. If you are unsure about your breathing pattern when you exercise, take a moment to compare your breathing pattern when not exercising versus when exercising. Notice the rate and depth of each. Here are a few warning signs that your breathing may no longer be asthma friendly:

If necessary, your GP or the A&E medical practitioner may replace the blue and grey reliever inhalers with a purple preventer device for aftercare. This may be repeated between two and seven days. Aftercare is crucial for managing asthma. If you have not been following a plan to stay healthy, your asthma may have started to deteriorate. In this case, you may need to switch to oral steroids (prednisone) until your condition improves. You should start taking oral corticosteroids before your appointment with the A&E or treatment room. You may not be able to retrieve your old medication, so it is important to pass on the necessary information to the medical practitioner. You may have stopped receiving your medication. If you require personal health assistance, make sure to have a bronchodilator as well as your reliever inhaler. Using a Puff Acceptor can help reduce inflammation. It is important to use it correctly in order to experience its benefits. Plain color should be used for the inhaler. Intranasal corticosteroids are only prescribed for specific purposes. If the current treatment is not sufficient, your doctor may add another remedy. Only four families have received creditable treatment so far. Plan your actions accordingly and make sure you know what steps to take.

Having a plan for emergencies is essential. It is important to be prepared for any potential issues that may arise, although they may not actually occur. In the event of an asthma attack during exercise, your doctor or another healthcare professional may provide you with a written emergency care plan. This plan will advise you on which medications to take if your asthma symptoms worsen. During an asthma attack, the blue and grey reliever inhalers (most likely Ventolin or Bricanyl) serve as a first aid. These medications work to open up your airways and provide relief for your asthma. If you feel that your asthma symptoms are worsening, take 2 puffs of your light brown or blue reliever inhaler immediately. If there is no improvement after the first puff, take the second puff after 5 minutes (or sooner for children). If there is still little or no change, take a third puff 5 minutes after the second puff. If your asthma symptoms do not improve or if they return, it is important to go to the Accident and Emergency Department of the nearest hospital immediately. A medical practitioner will be able to assist you as quickly as possible. If you have an individual action plan for your asthma, be sure to bring a copy of it to the A&E. Do not drive yourself to the A&E if your asthma medication has proven to be ineffective.

7. Creating an Asthma-Friendly Exercise Routine

Create a Plan: Set reasonable goals for yourself. The U.S. Department of Health and Human Services recommends at least 150 minutes a week of moderate-intensity exercise. Instead of devoting hours to physical fitness all at once, it may be easier to fit in small chunks of exercise throughout the day. For instance, a quick daily brisk walk can help you fit in your 150 minutes. As you begin to identify physical activities that are suited to both your abilities and your asthma, set out your exercise plan. Best-case scenario, phase in your workout routine gradually. Remember, it's completely normal for your physical fitness routine to change. It's also ideal to re-evaluate how you're doing every now and then and make changes accordingly. And you may want to consider doing this if you start to experience symptoms, such as coughing or wheezing, which could indicate that your asthma is flaring up.

Asthma attacks can be triggered by a variety of things, and for some people, physical activity can be a prime asthma trigger. If you're in this group, these general strategies and expert tips may help you create an asthmatic-friendly routine. Some researchers think that physical exercise can positively affect airway inflammation, making asthma symptoms less severe. Still, when starting a new exercise plan, your cheapest tools are a conversation with your doctor and a bit of research!

7.1. 1. Setting Realistic Goals

It is important to make sure the person goes at his or her pace and make sure they understand the goal is to become stronger, healthier and not necessarily reach a certain fitness level or be able to compete. Someone with asthma might have to start with walking and do a few minutes of yoga, until they are able to build up and progress, so people should be advised to set goals feasible to their ability to prevent getting discouraged and giving up. You have to start out small and gradually work your way up. Many asthma patients have developed the condition prior to exercising and they need to build up their lungs to take on more physical activity. If there was no previous exercise, an asthma patient needs to focus on the person's individual needs and health condition and to make sure precautions are considered regarding the severity of any attacks and when and where to exercise.

When it comes to setting a realistic goal for yourself or others, it is very important to make sure the individual understands their health status and is realistic about what they can and cannot do. Although it can also be motivating to see people change at 4 weeks when offered an exercise program, the importance is not the time period, but to improve. It is very rewarding for the patient to see the changes for themselves, but remember that rewards are only short-lived. If you do not meet your goals, it certainly does not work to reward yourself. It is helpful for some people to understand and weigh out the benefits of exercise versus not exercising, and how they manage symptoms as well as the asthma management medications. This may also lead to setting attainable goals for that individual.

7.2. 2. Tracking Your Progress

Your fitness and endurance levels can also improve with time, contributing to greater confidence or comfort with activities and therefore a shift in asthma friendliness. This shift may be noticeable in terms of moving longer, further, or more easily. Feeling changes take place can be very motivating and help plan exercise goals. Improvements over time may be noticeable in lessening or changing asthma symptoms, changes in fitness, or just in how you feel during exercise. These signs indicate that you are moving in the right direction with exercise that is becoming more tolerated for your asthma.

To help stay on top of changes, some people find that it is helpful to keep track of the specifics of mild asthma symptoms and how symptoms have changed since beginning to be more active. Other individuals may prefer not to interrupt their exercise with the recording of data or manage asthma in a way that exercise is always comfortable and somewhat easy. These decisions are based on individual preferences, personality, and personal asthma action plan in collaboration with a healthcare provider. Symptoms tracked can include: shortness of breath; how fast you become short of breath; and any changes in coughing, wheezing, sputum or chest problems.

Checking in on your progress is important for making sure you are on the right path to managing your asthma with exercise. Do the specifics of your symptoms or asthma differ since becoming more active? Are you able to move more easily or participate in activities longer than before? Or, have your energy levels, mood, or sleep quality changed? The answers to these questions provide you with valuable information to continue your journey of identifying the most asthma-friendly exercises for your unique self.

8. Conclusion and Final Recommendations

Final Recommendations In general, individuals should not avoid participating in exercise due to asthma. They should communicate with doctors and express their feelings. They should consult with exercise professionals to develop an appropriate exercise program. Personalized strategies based on an individual's condition(s), the exercises identified, and strategies that may need to enhance performance are necessary. Individuals with asthma should exercise at a level and type that is comfortable based on those aforementioned things and avoid their triggers. Finally, they should avoid exercising outside in cold air or high pollen seasons if those are triggers.

Conclusion This paper has explored the multifaceted intersections between asthma and physical activity in order to craft feasible, personalized strategies through which people with asthma can lead healthier, more active lives. Using a holistic lens, the paper defined asthma and the factors responsible for and affected by its development present in individuals; asthma and its influences on and relationship with physical activity; the world of exercise science and its recommendations; the experiences of individuals with asthma/asthma-related symptoms who would like to become more active; and finally, a detailed examination of beneficial exercises and exercises that may need to be adapted based on underlying physical condition(s). This paper argues for the creation of feasible exercise-induced bronchoconstriction (EIB)-free zones and spaces; definition of personal goals, equipment availability, and comfort for people with asthma providing advice and knowledge about different equipment regarding those two goals; looking at the spectrum of healthy to non-healthy individuals; and approaches to be mindful of for very physically active asthmatics, based on those recommendations.